Gluten Free

Christmas

Recipes

Laura Sommers is **The Recipe Lady!**

She is a loving wife and mother who lives on a small farm in Baltimore County, Maryland and has a passion for all things domestic especially when it comes to saving money. She has a profitable eBay business and is a couponing addict. Follow her tips and tricks to learn how to make delicious meals on a budget, save money or to learn the latest life hack!

Visit her Amazon Author Page to see her latest books:

amazon.com/author/laurasommers

Visit the Recipe Lady's blog for even more great recipes and to learn which books are **FREE** for download each week:

http://the-recipe-lady.blogspot.com/

Subscribe to The Recipe Lady blog through Amazon and have recipes and updates sent directly to your Kindle:

The Recipe Lady Blog through Amazon

Laura Sommers is also an Extreme Couponer and Penny Hauler! If you would like to find out how to get things for **FREE** with coupons or how to get things for only a **PENNY**, then visit her couponing blog **Penny Items and Freebies**

http://penny-items-and-freebies.blogspot.com/

Other Books by Laura Sommers

- **Gluten Free Baking Recipes**

- **Gluten Free Cookie Recipes**

- **Gluten Free Cauliflower Recipes**

- **Gluten Free Cake Recipes**

- **Gluten Free Bread Recipes**

Introduction

Eating gluten free needn't mean you have to suffer during Christmas! You can still enjoy the holidays but in a gluten free version! No sacrificing of taste.

Get the best gluten free Christmas recipes in this book!
Discover delicious gluten free bread recipes the whole family will love!
Great recipes for those with gluten intolerance, celiac disease, or who are eating a gluten-free diet for other reasons.

Each Gluten Free Christmas recipe in this cookbook is easy to prepare with step-by-step instructions. So if you have a wheat allergy or have gluten intolerance, there are many wonderful recipes in this book to give you lots and lots of options to enjoy!

Preventing Contamination

When you have a gluten or wheat allergy or you are just gluten intolerant, you have to be very careful about cross contamination, especially if others in your family don't share your quest for a gluten free life style. Here are some things to be aware of to prevent wheat products from accidentally getting in to your gluten free products.

Keep all you gluten free items in an air tight container.
Wash all surfaces thoroughly before making any gluten free products.
Ideally, have a separate work area or counter that is reserved for gluten free only items.
Have a separate cabinet for anything gluten free and have a strict rule that it is gluten free only!
Label all gluten free items clearly as Gluten Free.
Have a separate section of the refrigerator or a completely separate refrigerator if possible for all gluten free items.
Have your own container of butter or margarine. A very common culprit of cross contamination is someone buttering their wheat based toast with butter and then sticking the knife back in the butter or scraping the excess off the sides in to the tub of butter.
Have a separate toaster and keep it on a separate counter away from the "gluten toaster." Try to keep both toasters clean but away from each other.

Those are a few tips and tricks to help prevent cross contamination. I hope that they were helpful.

Gluten Free Gingerbread Cake

Ingredients:

1 cup amaranth flour
1 cup buckwheat flour
1/2 cup coconut flour
2 1/2 tsps. baking soda
2 tsps. ground cinnamon
2 tsps. ground ginger
1/2 tsp. ground cloves
1/2 tsp. ground nutmeg
1/2 tsp. salt
2 tbsps. flax seed meal
6 tbsps. water
3/4 cup agave nectar
3/4 cup canola oil
3/4 cup molasses
2 tsps. grated fresh ginger
1 tsp. lemon zest, or more to taste
1 cup boiling water

Directions:

1. Preheat oven to 350 degrees F (175 degrees C).
2. Grease a 9x13-inch baking pan.
3. Mix amaranth flour, buckwheat flour, coconut flour, baking soda, cinnamon, ground ginger, cloves, nutmeg, and salt together in a large bowl.
4. Make a well in the center of the flour mixture.
5. Stir flax meal and 6 tbsps. water together in a separate bowl.
6. Add agave nectar, canola oil, molasses, grated fresh ginger, and lemon zest; stir to combine.
7. Pour wet ingredients into the well in the flour mixture; mix well. Gradually stir boiling water into the batter until fully incorporated.
8. Pour batter into prepared baking pan.
9. Bake in the preheated oven until a toothpick inserted into the center of the cake comes out clean, 35 to 40 minutes.

Gluten-Free Cherry Crumble

Ingredients:

1/3 cup butter
3 cups pitted cherries
10 tbsps. white sugar, divided
2 tsps. lemon juice
1 cup gluten-free all-purpose baking flour
1 tsp. vanilla powder
1 tsp. ground nutmeg
1 tsp. ground cinnamon

Directions:

1. Cube butter and place in freezer until firm, about 15 minutes.
2. Preheat air fryer to 325 degrees F (165 degrees C).
3. Combine pitted cherries, 2 tbsps. sugar and lemon juice in a bowl; mix well.
4. Pour cherry mixture into baking dish.
5. Mix flour and 6 tbsps. of sugar in a bowl.
6. Cut in butter using fingers until particles are pea-size.
7. Distribute over cherries and press down lightly.
8. Stir 2 tbsps. sugar, vanilla powder, nutmeg, and cinnamon together in a bowl.
9. Dust sugar topping over the cherries and flour.
10. Bake in the preheated air fryer.
11. Check at 25 minutes; if not yet browned, continue cooking and checking at 5-minute intervals until slightly browned.
12. Close drawer and turn off air fryer.
13. Leave crumble inside for 10 minutes.
14. Remove and allow to cool slightly, about 5 minutes.

Gluten-Free Cherry Cobbler Muffins

Ingredients:

2 cups gluten-free all-purpose baking flour
1/2 cup white sugar
1 tsp. gluten-free baking powder
1 cup milk
1/4 cup vegetable oil
1 egg, beaten
1/2 tsp. vanilla extract
1/2 tsp. almond extract
2 cups pitted and chopped fresh cherries (including any juice from chopping)
Streusel Topping:
1/4 cup gluten-free rolled oats
1/4 cup brown sugar
1/4 cup white sugar
2 tbsps. cold butter, cut into pieces

Directions:

1. Preheat oven to 375 degrees F (190 degrees C).
2. Line 24 muffin cups with paper liners.
3. Mix flour, 1/2 cup sugar, and baking powder in a large bowl.
4. Whisk milk, vegetable oil, egg, vanilla extract, and almond extract together in a separate bowl.
5. Make a well in the center of the flour mixture; pour in milk mixture.
6. Stir until batter is just blended and slightly lumpy; gently fold in cherries and cherry juice.
7. Fill muffin cups 2/3 full with batter.
8. Mix oats, brown sugar, 1/4 cup white sugar, and butter together in a bowl until crumbly; sprinkle oat mixture over batter.
9. Bake in the preheated oven until a toothpick inserted in the center of a muffin comes out clean, about 20 minutes.

Gluten Free Gingerbread Drops

Ingredients:

1 1/2 cups canned pinto beans, drained and rinsed
2 tbsps. molasses
1 tbsp. oil
2 tbsps. rice flour
2 tbsps. amaranth
1/2 tsp. ground cinnamon
1/4 tsp. ground ginger
1/2 cup raisin

Directions:

1. Preheat oven to 375 degrees F (190 degrees C).
2. Line a baking sheet with parchment paper.
3. Mash beans, molasses, and oil together in a bowl using a potato masher or fork.
4. Stir rice flour, amaranth, cinnamon, and ginger into bean mixture until dough is well combined; fold in raisins.
5. Form dough into 24 small balls and arrange on prepared baking sheet. Slightly flatten balls onto baking sheet.
6. Bake in the preheated oven until edges are slightly hardened, 12 to 14 minutes.
7. Cool on baking sheet for 2 minutes before transferring to a wire rack.

Gluten Free Eggnog

Ingredients:

Ice
Cold water
6 large eggs
1 cup granulated sugar
4 cups whole milk
1 tsp. vanilla extract
1/2 tsp. ground nutmeg

Directions:

1. In a large bowl, combine ice and cold water. Bowl should be large enough to place your saucepan without having the ice and water slop over the sides and into your cooked eggnog.
2. In small bowl, whisk together eggs, 1/2 the granulated sugar, and 1 cup of the milk. Combine remaining milk and sugar in a heavy-bottomed 4 quart pot.
3. Bring milk to a boil over medium high heat. Reduce heat to low and slowly whisk one cup of hot milk into the egg mixture.
4. In a slow and steady stream, whisk egg mixture into the hot milk. Increase heat to medium.
5. Cook, whisking constantly, until mixture reaches 185 degrees F.
6. Eggnog should thicken and coat the back of a wooden spoon.
7. Immediately place pot into the ice bath and whisk until cool.
8. Add vanilla and nutmeg. Transfer to a covered container and chill overnight.
9. Serve with a little nutmeg sprinkled onto of the eggnog, if desired.
10. Serve with a splash of bourbon or your favorite adult spirit.

Gluten Free Eggnog Cupcakes

Ingredients:

1 cup gluten free flour blend (add 1 tsp. xanthan gum if your blend doesn't have it.)
1/2 cup almond flour
3/4 cup sugar
1 tsp. baking powder
1/2 tsp. baking soda
1/4 tsp. nutmeg
1 tsp. cinnamon
1/2 cup eggnog
1/2 cup butter melted
2 large eggs
1 dash salt
For Icing:
1 1/4 cup powdered sugar
2 tbsps. eggnog
1/4 tsp. cinnamon
1/8 tsp. nutmeg

Directions:

1. Preheat the oven to 350 degrees F.
2. In a mixer, add all wet ingredients.
3. Slowly add in dry ingredients while beating on medium high speed.
4. Line a muffin tin with paper cupcake liners.
5. Use a soup scoop to pour batter into each, so they are about 3/4 full.
6. Bake for 20 minutes.
7. Remove and put on a cooling rack.

Icing Directions:

1. Put powdered sugar into a mixer. Power it on low and add eggnog.
2. Turn the speed up until the icing is whipped.
3. Spread onto cupcakes when they are cool.

Gluten-Free Chocolate Chip Cookies

Ingredients:

1 med. banana
1 cup peanut butter
1 egg
1 tsp. vanilla
1/2 tsp. baking soda
1/2 cup sugar
1/4 tsp. salt
1 1/2 cup semisweet chocolate chips

Directions:

1. Preheat oven to 350 degrees F.
2. Mash banana in a large mixing bowl.
3. Add peanut butter, egg, vanilla, baking soda, sugar and salt, stirring to combine.
4. Fold in chocolate chips.
5. Drop heaping spoonfuls of dough on a parchment-lined baking sheet, placing cookies about 1 1/2" apart.
6. Bake for 9-10 minutes, or until cookies are lightly golden.

Gluten Free Coconut Christmas Sugar Stars

Ingredients:

1.5 cups gluten free flour
1.5 tsps. psyllium husk powder
1/2 tsp. cream of tartar
1/2 tsp. baking soda
1/8 tsp. salt
1/2 cup organic shortening
1/2 cup coconut sugar
1/4 cup coconut milk
2 tsps. pure vanilla extract

Directions:

1. Preheat oven to 350 degrees. Line two cookie sheets with parchment paper.
2. In a medium bowl, combine: gf flour, psyllium powder, cream of tartar, baking soda, and salt.
3. Cut in shortening.
4. In a separate cup, combine: sugar, milk, and vanilla.
5. Add to flour mixture and blend thoroughly. Add a tsp. or two of water if dough is too dry.
6. Gather dough into a ball and refrigerate for a few minutes until slightly chilled.
7. Roll dough out between layers of parchment paper.
8. Peel top layer of parchment off and cut into shapes.
9. Depending on how warm the dough is, you may want to chill the dough again.
10. Use a spatula to transfer cookies to a parchment lined cookie sheet.
11. Brush unbaked cookies with water before sprinkling with vegan cane or coconut sugar.
12. Bake time will vary, depending on size and thickness of dough.
13. Small 2-inch stars bake for 9-10 minutes.

Gluten Free Chocolate Christmas Truffles

Ingredients:

2/3 cup avocado mashed. (about 1 large)
1/4 cup + 2 tbsp. unsweetened cocoa powder
1/2 tsp vanilla extract
1 tsp almond extract omit if you just want straight up chocolate
2/3 cup milk chocolate chips
1/2 cup sweetened coconut flakes

Directions:

1. Blend the avocado in a food processor until it is very smooth.
2. Add in the protein powder, vanilla extract and almond extract and blend until well combined.
3. In a medium, microwave safe bowl microwave the chocolate chips for about 1 1/2 minutes, stirring every 20 seconds, until the chips are melted.
4. Add the avocado mixture into the bowl of melted chocolate and stir very well until the chocolate is mixed well.
5. Cover the bowl with saran wrap and refrigerate for 2 hours.
6. Line a cookie sheet with waxed paper, and place the sweetened coconut flakes in shallow plate.
7. Using a small cookie scoop the scoop the mixture and roll around in your hands to create even balls.
8. Roll each ball around in the coconut flakes and place on the prepared cookie sheet.
9. Keep in the refrigerator until ready to serve.

Gluten Free Gingerbread Men

Ingredients:

2 1/2 cups almond flour
1/3 cup ground flaxseed
1/2 tsp. baking soda
2 tbsps. ground ginger
1 tsp. fresh ginger, grated
1 1/2 tsps. cinnamon
1/2 tsp. ground nutmeg
1/2 tsp. ground cloves
1/2 tsp. vanilla powder
1/4 cup coconut oil, melted
1/4 cup honey
1 egg, lightly beaten
1/3 cup white chocolate, melted

Directions:

1. Combine almond flour, flax seed, baking soda, ground ginger, fresh ginger, cinnamon, nutmeg, cloves and vanilla powder in a large mixing bowl and stir until well combined
2. Add coconut oil, honey and egg to the bowl with the dry ingredients and mix until well combined
3. Roll mixture into a ball and wrap in cling film.
4. Put in freezer for 30 minutes and then transfer to fridge for another 30 minutes
5. Remove the dough from the cling film and place between two large pieces of baking paper. With a rolling pin roll the dough out to around 3mm thick
6. With a gingerbread cookie cutter, cut into shapes.
7. The dough is delicate so it is best to remove the remaining dough from the outside of the cut out cookie and take a sharp knife or metal spatula under the cookie and carefully place on a tray lined with baking paper
8. Bake for 10 minutes or until golden.
9. They should still be slightly soft when they come out of the oven
10. Allow the cookies to completely cool
11. Melt the white chocolate and add to a piping bag with a thin nozzle.
12. Pipe on the chocolate to decorate the cookies with your favorite design

Gluten Free Sweet Potato Pie

Crust Ingredients:

1 cup almond flour
1 cup coconut flour
2 tbsp. tapioca starch
1/2 tsp. salt
3 tbsps. olive oil*
8 tbsps. ice water
1 egg lightly beaten

Filling Ingredients:

3 cups small sweet potatoes
1-1/2 sweet potato puree
2 eggs
1/4 cup unsweetened almond milk
1/3 cup honey
1/4 tsp. cardamom
1 tsp. ground cinnamon
1/4 tsp. ground corriander
1/4 tsp. ground ginger
1/8 tsp. ground cloves
1 tsp. pure vanilla extract
1 tsp. lemon juice
1/2 tsp. salt

Crust Directions:

1. Add almond flour, coconut flour, tapioca starch and salt to a food processor.
2. Pulse flour until combined and any chunks are smoothed out.
3. Begin adding oil and water one tbsp. at a time, continuing to pulse between tbsps.
4. First, beads the size of peas should form and as you add, dough should begin coming together
5. Once you have added all the oil and water, add the lightly beaten egg.
6. Dough should come together in one big hunk.
7. Take the dough in your hands and smoosh it into a ball, then form a disk.
8. Wrap tightly in plastic wrap and freeze for at least 2 hours.

Pie Directions:

1. Poke holes in the sweet potatoes using a fork and roast for 40 to 50 minutes 400 degrees in the oven.
2. Allow sweet potatoes to cool enough to handle.
3. The skin should peel away from the flesh easily.
4. Remove skin and discard.
5. Heat the oven to 400 degrees.
6. Place flesh in a blender along with the rest of the filling ingredients. Blend until completely smooth.
7. Remove pie crust from refrigerator.
8. Roll out half of the pie crust or smoosh it with your fingers into a pie dish (use the other half for another sweet potato pie).
9. Pour sweet potato mixture into the pie crust and smooth with a spatula.
10. Bake in the oven for 10 minutes at 400 degrees then lower the temperature to 325 and bake an additional 30 minutes, until pie does not jiggle when shaken.
11. Allow pie to cool at least one hour before serving.
12. You can chill the pie in the refrigerator and serve it cold.

Gluten Free Cranberry White Chocolate Pecan Cookies

Ingredients:

3/4 cup dried sweetened cranberries
1 tsp. vanilla extract
2 eggs , lightly beaten
1 stick unsalted butter, softened
1/2 cup granulated Sugar
1/4 cup light brown sugar
1 3/4 cup gluten free oat flour
½ tsp. baking powder
½ tsp. kosher salt
½ tsp. ground cinnamon
½ cup pecan halves , rough chopped
1 cup white chocolate*

Directions:

1. In a small mixing bowl, combine the cranberries, eggs and vanilla.
2. Cover with plastic wrap and allow to sit at room temperature for 30 minutes.
3. In a mixing bowl, cream the butter.
4. Add the granulated and brown sugar and cream together.
5. In a separate mixing bowl, combine the oat flour, baking powder, salt and cinnamon.
6. With the mixer running on low, pour in the dry ingredients and fully mix together (the mixture will be dry).
7. Pour in the cranberry-egg mixture and mix until fully combined. Mix in the pecans and white chocolate just until incorporated; do not over mix.
8. Place the dough, covered with plastic wrap into the refrigerator for 2 hours.
9. Preheat oven to 350 degrees. Using a small dining spoon, scoop a spoonful onto a silpat or parchment-lined baking sheet, form loosely into a ball shape (do not overwork the dough).
10. Bake for 13 minutes or until the bottom begins to turn dark golden brown. Remove from oven, allow to sit on cookie sheet for 5 minutes. Remove and let cool fully on a cooling rack.

Gluten Free Cranberry Bread

Ingredients:

6 tbsps. unsalted butter, at room temperature
1 cup granulated sugar, plus 1 tbsp.
2 eggs at room temperature, beaten
2 1/2 cups all-purpose gluten-free flour
1 tsp. xanthan gum (omit if your blend already contains it)
1 tsp. baking powder
1/2 tsp. baking soda
3/4 tsp. kosher salt
10 oz. fresh cranberries, halved
1/2 cup milk, at room temperature*
1/2 cup sour cream, at room temperature

Directions:

1. Preheat your oven to 350 degrees F. Grease or line a standard 9 x 5-inch loaf pan and set it aside.
2. In the bowl of a stand mixer fitted with the paddle attachment, or a large bowl with a handheld mixer, place the butter.
3. Beat on medium-high speed until light and fluffy.
4. Add the 1 cup of granulated sugar and the eggs, beating well after each addition.
5. In a separate, medium-size bowl, place the flour blend, xanthan gum, baking powder, baking soda and salt, and whisk to combine well.
6. Place the cranberry halves in a separate, small bowl.
7. Add about one tbsp. of the dry ingredients to the cranberries, and toss to coat.
8. Set the cranberries aside.
9. To the bowl with the butter and sugar mixture, add the dry ingredients, alternating with the milk and sour cream, beginning and ending with the dry ingredients.
10. The mixture will be thick but smooth. Add the cranberries and reserved dry ingredients, and mix gently into the batter until evenly distributed throughout.
11. Scrape the batter into the prepared pan, and smooth the top. It will nearly fill the pan.
12. Smooth the top with a wet spatula, and sprinkle with the remaining tbsp. of sugar.

13. Place the pan in the center of the preheated oven and bake, rotating once, until golden brown on top and a toothpick inserted in the center comes out clean (about 1 hour).
14. Remove from the oven and allow to cool in the pan for 20 minutes before transferring to a wire rack to cool completely.
15. Slice and serve.

Gluten Free Cranberry Sauce

Ingredients:

12 oz. fresh cranberries
3/4 cup fresh orange juice
1/2 cup honey

Directions:

1. Combine cranberries, orange juice, and honey in sauce pan.
2. Simmer over medium heat, until berries pop and sauce thickens, about 10 - 15 minutes.
3. Cool completely and refrigerate.
4. Serve at room temperature.

Gluten Free Christmas Cranberry Lemon Cake

Ingredients:

1 1/4 cups fresh cranberries
1 tbsp. of sugar, plus additional 3/4 cup
1 cup gluten free flour mix
1 1/4 tsp baking powder
1/2 tsp salt
6 tbsp. unsalted butter (3/4 of a stick)
1/2 cup whole milk (can substitute light cream), at room temp if possible
1 tsp vanilla extract
1 egg
Zest of 1 lemon (about 2 tsp.)

Directions:

1. Preheat oven to 350 degrees.
2. Coat a 9-inch cake pan or dish with cooking spray.
3. In a small bowl, toss cranberries with 1 tbsp. of the sugar.
4. Set aside.
5. In a large bowl, whisk together the flour, remaining 3/4 cup of sugar, baking powder, and salt.
6. In another bowl or dish, melt the butter in the microwave.
7. Add the milk and vanilla, and whisk to combine.
8. Add the egg and whisk once more.
9. If the mixture seizes up (because the milk was too cold) just pop it in the microwave for 10 seconds at a time until the mixture is a liquid.
10. Pour the liquid ingredients into the large bowl with the dry ingredients, and whisk to combine. Add the lemon zest to the batter and whisk again.
11. Pour the batter into the greased cake pan and, if necessary, spread evenly with a rubber spatula. Scatter the sugared cranberries over the top. Sprinkle any excess sugar on top of the cake.
12. Bake for 30 to 35 minutes, until the middle of the cake only jiggles slightly. Allow the cake to cool for at least 20 minutes before slicing.

Gluten Free Stained Glass Cookies

Ingredients:

1.5 sticks dairy free margarine, or butter
1 cup sugar
2 large eggs
3.5 cups all purpose gluten free flour blend
1 tsp. xanthan gum omit if included in your flour blend
1 tsp. gluten free baking powder
1/2 tsp. vanilla extract
1/2 tsp. almond extract
1 lb. bag of hard clear candies like Jolly Ranchers

Directions:

1. You will need two cookies cutters of the same shape, with one smaller than the other for the cut out centers.
2. Preheat your oven to 350 degrees F
3. Separate the hard candies into their various colors and put each color in a small ziplock bag.
4. Using a rolling pin or something similar carefully smash the candies into small pieces.
5. Cream together margarine and sugar.
6. Add in eggs and vanilla and almond extracts and mix until combined, remember to scrape down the sides of the bowl.
7. Measure out the dry ingredients into another bowl and mix by hand to combine the gum and baking powder.
8. Add the dry ingredients to the sugar and egg mixture and mix well to combine.
9. If the cookie dough is too soft to roll out at this point, place it in a bag or in a covered bowl in the fridge to allow the margarine to harden enough so that you can roll it out later.
10. When the dough has hardened roll it out on parchment paper, I use cling wrap to cover the top of the dough as I roll it out so that it does not stick to the rolling pin, I don't use extra flour.
11. Transfer the cut out cookies to the lined baking sheet and then use a smaller cutter with the same shape to cut out the centers.
12. Fill the center of the cookies with approximately 1/2 to 1 tsp crushed candy.
13. Bake cookies for 12 - 14 minutes at 350 degrees F on a parchment lined baking sheet.

14. Allow to cool on baking sheet, the cookies will firm up once cooled and the 'glass' center will harden.
15. The candy will be bubbling when it comes out of the oven, this is normal and it will spread out when it cools down and the bubbles should disappear.

Gluten Free Chewy Christmas Thumbprint Cookies

Ingredients:

2 cups blanched almond flour
1/4 cup coconut flour, sifted if lumpy
1/2 cup raw or granulated sugar
1 tsp. baking powder
1/8 tsp. salt
7 tbsps. coconut oil, melted and cooled slightly
1 large egg, room temperature
1 tsp. almond extract
1/3 cup raspberry jam
1/2 cup white chocolate for piping

Directions:

1. In a medium bowl, stir together the almond flour, coconut flour, sugar, baking powder and salt.
2. In another medium bowl, stir together the coconut oil, egg and almond extract.
3. Add the flour mixture to the wet mixture and stir just until combined.
4. The dough will feel quite wet. Let sit for 10 minutes, which allows the coconut flour to absorb the liquid.
5. Preheat the oven to 350 °F (175 °C) and line a cookie sheet with a piece of parchment paper.
6. Roll the dough into 1" balls and place 2" apart on the prepared cookie sheet. The dough will feel quite greasy but this is okay.
7. Using your thumb, make an indentation about 3/4 of the way down into each cookie.
8. You may want to re-form the edges a little to make them prettier.
9. Fill each indentation with 1/2 tsp. of jam.
10. Be sure not to overfill them.
11. Bake for 8 minutes or until the cookies have barely started browning on the bottom.
12. Let the cookies, which will be very soft, cool for 5 minutes on the baking sheet and then remove to a wire rack to cool completely.
13. Pipe with white chocolate, if desired.
14. Refrigerate in an airtight container for up to 4 days.

Gluten Free Frosted Sugar Cookies

Cookie Ingredients:

1 cup shortening
1 cup granulated sugar
1 large eggs, cold
1 tbsp. vanilla extract
3 cup gluten free all-purpose flour, plus more for rolling out the dough
1 tsp. fine sea salt

Frosting Ingredients:

1/2 cup vegan butter
1/2 cup vegetable shortening
3 cup powdered sugar
1 tsp. vanilla extract
2 tbsp. unsweetened coconut milk
food coloring, optional
gluten free sprinkles

Cookie Directions:

1. Preheat oven to 350 degrees F and line baking sheets with silicon mats or parchment paper.
2. In the bowl of a stand mixer, cream together the shortening and sugar until light and creamy, about 1-2 minutes.
3. Mix in the egg and the vanilla extract.
4. Add the flour and salt and mix on low speed until completely incorporated.
5. The dough should be slightly firm but still pliable - not sticky, and not too stiff.
6. Turn half of the the dough out onto floured parchment paper.
7. Cover with plastic wrap and roll out until it's about 1/4 inch thick.
8. Use desired cookie cutters to cut into shapes.
9. Repeat with the remaining dough. Dough scraps can be re-rolled.
10. Transfer the cookies (carefully) to the prepared baking pans and bake 8-10 minutes (mine were done in 9 but it will depend on the size of your cookie cutters and thickness of your dough).
11. Cool cookies on the baking sheet for a few minutes before cooling completely on a wire rack.
12. Bake cookies in batches if necessary.
13. Cool completely before frosting.

Frosting Directions:

1. Add the shortening, vegan butter, and powdered sugar to the bowl of a stand mixer.
2. Mix on low speed until the sugar is incorporated.
3. Turn the mixer to medium-high and beat for 1 minute.
4. Mix in the vanilla extract and milk and mix until the frosting is light and fluffy, about 1 minute or less.
5. Mix in food coloring if using.
6. Frost the cookies and top with sprinkles.
7. Serve immediately or store in an airtight container until ready to serve.

Gluten-Free Green Bean Casserole

Ingredients:

1 can (18 oz) cream of mushroom soup
1 tsp. gluten free soy sauce
Dash ground black pepper
2 tbsps. gluten free plain bread crumbs
2 bags (12 oz. each) frozen cut green beans, thawed

Directions:

Heat oven to 350 degrees F.
In ungreased 1 1/2-quart casserole, mix soup, soy sauce, pepper, bread crumbs and green beans.
Bake about 40 minutes or until hot and bubbly.

Gluten Free Stuffing

Ingredients:

1 (1 lb.) loaf gluten-free bread
3 tbsps. olive oil
2 onions, diced
3 stalks celery, diced
1 tsp. chopped fresh sage
1 tsp. dried thyme leaves
3/4 tsp.
Salt ground black pepper to taste
2 cups gluten-free chicken broth
2 large eggs

Directions:

1. Preheat oven to 325 degrees F (165 degrees C).
2. Grease a 3-quart baking dish.
3. Cut bread into cubes about 3/4-inch square and spread onto a baking sheet.
4. Bake in the preheated oven until crisp, 12 to 17 minutes.
5. Heat olive oil in a large skillet over medium heat.
6. Cook and stir onions and celery in the hot oil until soft, 8 to 10 minutes.
7. Stir sage, thyme, salt, and black pepper into the vegetables.
8. Mix toasted bread crumbs, chicken broth, and eggs into vegetables.
9. Spoon dressing into the prepared baking dish and cover dish.
10. Bake in the preheated oven for 30 minutes, uncover, and bake until top of dressing is crisp and lightly browned, about 10 more minutes.

Gluten Free Gravy

Ingredients:

5 tbsps. turkey fat, unsalted butter, or olive oil
5 tbsps. sweet rice flour
1 quart chicken or turkey stock, divided
1/2 cup skimmed roasting pan juices
Kosher salt
Freshly ground black pepper
1 tsp. tamari
Minced fresh herbs like thyme, rosemary, or sage

Directions:

1. Make a gluten-free roux: Heat the fat over medium-low heat in a small saucepan until shimmering. Sprinkle in the flour.
2. When it hits the fat, it will be very thick. After 30 seconds or so, the mixture relaxes into a creamy, bubbling paste. Whisk constantly during this process to keep the roux from burning.
3. Cook, whisking constantly, until golden-brown, 2 to 4 minutes.
4. Whisk in 1 cup of the stock.
5. Cook, whisking constantly, until smooth.
6. Add the remaining 3 cups stock in a slow and steady stream.
7. For a thicker gravy, add only 2 to 2 1/2 cups of stock.
8. Cook the gravy until it gently bubbles and thickens, about 5 minutes.
9. Stir in pan juices, if using.
10. Season with salt and pepper as needed.
11. Add the additional seasonings as desired.

Gluten-Free Cornbread and Mushroom Stuffing

Ingredients:

8 cups day-old, gluten-free cornbread cubes (about 1 inch in diameter)
1/2 cup pecans, coarsely chopped
Cooking spray or butter
4 tbsps. unsalted butter
1 large onion, diced
3 medium celery ribs, thinly sliced crosswise
2 cloves garlic, minced
2 tsps. fresh rosemary leaves, coarsely chopped
1 tsp. fresh thyme leaves
1 tsp. kosher salt
1/4 tsp. freshly ground black pepper
1 lb. mixed fresh mushrooms, such as cremini, shiitake, and oyster, stems removed and coarsely chopped
1/2 cup dry white wine
2 large eggs, lightly beaten
2 cups low-sodium chicken or vegetable broth

Directions:

1. Arrange a rack in the middle of the oven and heat to 350 degrees F.
2. Divide the cubed cornbread onto 2 baking sheets and spread in an even layer.
3. Toast in the oven for 10 minutes.
4. Stir the bread and divide the pecans among the two baking sheets.
5. Bake until the bread is completely dry and the pecans are toasted, about 5 minutes more.
6. Remove the baking sheets from the oven and let cool.
7. Increase the oven temperature to 375°F. Grease a 9x13-inch baking dish with butter or cooking spray.
8. Melt the 4 tbsps. butter in a large skillet over medium heat.
9. Add the onion and celery and cook until softened, 6 to 8 minutes.
10. Stir in the garlic, rosemary, thyme, salt, and pepper, and cook for 1 minute.
11. Add the mushrooms and cook until slightly softened, about 5 minutes.
12. Pour in the wine, and cook until it's mostly reduced.
13. Remove the pan from the heat.

14. Place the bread, nuts, and mushroom mixture in a large bowl and stir to combine. Stir in the eggs.
15. Slowly pour the broth over the stuffing mixture, stirring as you go, so that the bread is well-coated and moistened.
16. Transfer the stuffing to the prepared baking dish.
17. Cover tightly with aluminum foil and bake for 20 minutes.
18. Uncover and bake until the center is just set and the stuffing is golden-brown, about 20 minutes more.
19. Let the stuffing cool for about 10 minutes before serving.

Gluten Free Turkey

Ingredients:

1 turkey, any size
2 cups chicken or turkey broth
2 sticks (1 cup) unsalted butter, melted, for basting (optional)
Equipment:
Roasting pan (or an alternative roasting dish)
Roasting rack (or something to lift the turkey off the pan)
Turkey baster, brush, or ladle (optional, if basting)

Directions:

1. Prepare the turkey for roasting. 30 minutes to 1 hour before roasting.
2. Take the turkey out of the refrigerator.
3. Remove any packaging and the bag of giblets.
4. Set the turkey breast-side up on a roasting rack and let it sit while the oven preheats.
5. Preheat the oven to 450 degrees F.
6. Position an oven rack in the bottom third of the oven, remove any racks above it, and heat to 450 degrees F.
7. Add liquid to the roasting pan.
8. When ready to roast, pour the broth or water into a roasting pan.
9. Place the turkey in the oven and immediately turn down the heat to 350 degrees F.
10. Roast the turkey. The rule of thumb for cooking a turkey is 13 minutes per pound. So our 16-pound turkey was estimated to cook in about 3 1/2 hours. However, some factors like brining the bird, cooking with an empty cavity, and leaving the legs un-trussed will contribute to much faster cooking.
11. Plan on the 13-minute-per-pound rule, but start checking the temperature of your turkey about halfway through the scheduled cooking time to gauge how fast it's cooking.
12. Every 45 minutes, remove the turkey from the oven, close the oven door, and baste the turkey all over.
13. In the last 45 minutes or so of cooking, you can also baste the turkey with melted butter or oil. This helps crisp up the skin and turn it a beautiful deep golden brown.
14. If your turkey is getting too browned, shield the breast meat loosely with aluminum foil toward the end of cooking.

15. Begin checking the turkey's temperature about halfway through the estimated cooking time. Check the temperature in 3 places: the breast, outer thigh, and inside thigh.
16. In every case, the meat should be at least 165 degrees F when the turkey has finished cooking.
17. If any place is under that temperature, put the turkey back in the oven for another 20 minutes.
18. Shield the breast meat with foil if needed to keep it from overcooking.
19. Rest the turkey before carving.
20. Grab one side of the roasting rack with an oven mitt and tilt the whole pan so the liquids inside the turkey cavity run out into the pan.
21. Then, lift the whole turkey (still on the rack) and transfer it to a cutting board.
22. Tent the turkey with aluminum foil and let it rest for at least 30 minutes. This gives time for the meat to firm up and the juices to be re-absorbed into the muscle tissue, making the turkey easier to slice and taste juicier.
23. Carve the turkey the same way you would carve a chicken.
24. Remove the wings first, then the thighs, then the breast meat.
25. Once you have the meat off, you can separate the thighs into thighs and drumsticks and carve the breast meat into individual slices.

Gluten Free Scalloped Potatoes

Ingredients:

2 tbsps. unsalted butter
1 medium onion, thinly sliced
4 cups whole milk
2 to 3 garlic cloves, smashed
1 heaping tsp. Dijon mustard
2 1/2 pounds (about 6 medium) baking potatoes, peeled
1 1/2 cups grated cheddar cheese, divided
3/4 cup heavy cream
Kosher salt and freshly ground black pepper

Directions:

1. Preheat oven to 375 degrees F.
2. Lightly grease a medium sized (1-1/2 to 2 quart) gratin or baking dish.
3. In a large Dutch oven, melt the butter over medium heat.
4. Add onions and sauté until softened, about 5 minutes.
5. Add the milk (or milk and water), garlic, and Dijon mustard and bring to a gentle boil over medium heat.
6. Add a generous amount of salt and pepper.
7. Meanwhile, slice the potatoes to 1/8-inch thickness, using a food processor or mandoline for even thickness. (Do not rinse the potatoes.) Add the potatoes to the milk and allow to simmer until the potatoes are almost tender — they should still have some resistance when poked with a paring knife — about 10 minutes.
8. Using a slotted spoon, transfer half of the potatoes and onions to the baking dish. (Discard the milk or save for another culinary use.)
9. Season generously with salt and pepper and top with 3/4 cup cheddar cheese.
10. Cover with the remaining potato mixture, season again with salt and pepper and top with remaining cheese. Pour the cream evenly over the potatoes and cheese.
11. Bake until crisp and golden on top, 50 minutes to 1 hour.
12. Allow to cool for at least 10 minutes before serving. (Leftovers make a perfect breakfast side.)

Gluten-Free Dinner Rolls

Ingredients:

3/4 cup warm (about 110°F) water
1 packet (2 tsps.) instant/rapid-rise yeast
2 cups millet flour
3/4 cup tapioca starch
2 tbsps. granulated sugar
2 tsps. xanthan gum
1 tsp. fine salt
1/2 tsp. baking powder
3 large eggs, lightly beaten
2 tbsps. olive or vegetable oil
1 tsp. apple cider vinegar

Directions:

1. Whisk the water and yeast together in a small bowl.
2. Allow to stand for about 3 minutes to dissolve.
3. In the bowl of a stand mixer, whisk together the millet flour, tapioca starch, sugar, xanthan gum, salt, and baking powder.
4. Fit the stand mixer with the paddle attachment.
5. Add the wet ingredients:
6. Add the yeast mixture, eggs, oil, and vinegar.
7. Beat on medium speed until a smooth batter forms, about 1 minute.
8. Without gluten to hold everything together, gluten-free yeast dough doesn't look anything like traditional wheat dough.
9. It looks more like a very thick cake batter.
10. Since the dough is so thick, it's best to mix it with a stand mixer.
11. Use the paddle attachment, not the dough hook, for this job. The dough won't form a cohesive ball. It should look like a smooth, thick cake batter.
12. Line a rimmed baking sheet with parchment paper. Drop dough, about 1/2 cup each, onto the baking sheet.
13. Cover the pan with a greased piece of plastic wrap. Allow dough to rise until light and puffy, about 45 minutes.
14. Preheat oven to 375°F. Uncover and bake until the rolls are golden-brown, about 15 minutes.
15. Remove pan from the oven and move the rolls to a cooling rack. Cool the rolls for at least 10 minutes before serving.

Gluten Free Pumpkin Pie

Ingredients:

1 (15-oz.) can pumpkin purée (not pumpkin pie filling)
1 tsp. vanilla extract
1 tsp. ground cinnamon
1/4 tsp. ground cloves
1/4 tsp. ground ginger
1/4 tsp. ground nutmeg
1/8 tsp. ground allspice
1 9-inch gluten-free pie crust
White rice flour, for dusting
1/2 cup packed light brown sugar
1 cup half and half, or full-fat coconut milk whisked until smooth
2 large eggs
1 large egg yolk
1/2 tsp. fine salt

Directions:

1. Arrange a rack in the middle of the oven and heat to 350 degrees F.
2. Purée the pumpkin purée with an immersion blender or in a food processor fitted with a blade attachment until smooth.
3. Spread the purée in an 8-inch square baking pan. Bake until the purée bubbles gently and turns slightly darker, about 18 minutes.
4. Remove the purée from the oven and transfer to a small bowl.
5. Stir in the vanilla, cinnamon, cloves, ginger, nutmeg, and allspice. Cover and refrigerate overnight.
6. Roll out the pie crust between two pieces of lightly white rice-floured parchment paper.
7. Remove the top piece of parchment and invert a 9-inch pie plate onto the center of the dough.
8. Slide your hand between the parchment and your counter.
9. Place your other hand on the back of the 9-inch pie plate. In one quick motion, flip the dough and pan over.
10. Press the dough into the pan. Slowly pull off the parchment paper. If the dough tore or ripped, press it back together. Trim and crimp the edges.
11. Chill for 20 minutes while the oven preheats.
12. Arrange a rack in the middle of the oven and heat to 400°F.
13. Line the pie crust with aluminum foil and fill with dried beans.
14. Bake until the edges just start to brown, about 12 to 15 minutes.
15. Remove the weights and foil.

16. Return the pan to the oven and bake for another 5 minutes.
17. Set the crust aside.
18. Reduce the oven temperature to 350 degrees F.
19. In a large bowl, whisk together the spiced pumpkin purée with the brown sugar until smooth.
20. Add the half-and-half or coconut milk, eggs, egg yolk, and salt.
21. Whisk until smooth. Place the pre-baked pie crust on a rimmed baking sheet and pour the filling into the pie crust.
22. Bake until set and a very light golden brown, about 40 minutes.
23. If the crust darkens too much before the filling has baked, cover the edges of the crust with foil to keep it from darkening.
24. The filling will jiggle slightly when you move the pan, but shouldn't look thin.
25. Remove from the oven and allow to cool before serving.

Gluten-Free Pie Crust

Ingredients:

2 1/2 cups millet flour
1/2 cup tapioca starch
1 tbsp. granulated sugar
1 1/2 tsps. xanthan gum
1/2 tsp. fine salt
1 cup (8 oz.) unsalted butter, shortening, or leaf lard, cold and cut into 16 pieces
6 to 8 tbsps. cold water, divided
White rice flour, for rolling

Directions:

1. Whisk the millet flour, tapioca starch, granulated sugar, xanthan gum, and salt together in a large bowl.
2. Cut in the fat with a pastry cutter until no large pieces of butter remain. The mixture should look coarse, with pieces of butter no larger than a pea.
3. Add 6 tbsps. of the water.
4. Stir with a wooden spoon until it just holds together. If the dough seems dry, add additional water 1 tbsp. at a time.
5. Dust a work surface with white rice flour. Divide the dough in half and pat each half into a disk. Wrap each disk well with plastic wrap and chill for 2 hours.
6. Remove the pie dough from the refrigerator and allow to sit out for about 10 minutes before rolling.
7. Sandwich the dough between parchment paper: Place a 13x18-inch piece of parchment paper on a work surface and lightly dust with white rice flour. Place a piece of dough on the center of the parchment and sprinkle with a little more flour. Cover the dough with the second piece of parchment paper.
8. Roll the dough from the center to edges, rotating the dough about a quarter of a turn after each roll. This keeps the dough round. Roll the crust about 2 inches larger than the bottom diameter of your pan. (For a 9-inch pie pan, roll the out into an 11-inch circle. This allows for enough dough to cover the sides of the pan.)
9. Remove the top piece of parchment from the dough. Invert the pie plate onto the center of the dough. Slide your hand between the bottom sheet of parchment paper and your counter. Place your other hand firmly on the back of the pie plate.

10. In one swift motion, flip the dough and plate. Gently press the dough into the edges of the plate and then slowly pull off the top piece of parchment.
11. Repair any cracks. If any part of the dough cracked or ripped, gently press it back together. Trim the edges of the crust.
12. Crimp the edges with a fork if desired. (This is for a single-crust pie.
13. For a double-crust pie, see Recipe Notes below.)
14. Chill the crust for 15 minutes before baking.

Gluten Free Mashed Potatoes

Ingredients:

4 large potatoes (about 3 pounds), peeled and quartered
1 medium onion, chopped
1 package (8 oz.) fat-free cream cheese, cubed
1 cup fat-free milk
1-1/4 tsps. salt
1/4 tsp. pepper

Directions:

1. Place potatoes and onion in a large saucepan and cover with water.
2. Bring to a boil. Reduce heat.
3. Cover and simmer for 15-20 minutes or until tender. Drain.
4. Transfer to a large bowl.
5. Add the cream cheese, milk, salt and pepper; beat until fluffy.

Gluten Free Sweet Potato Casserole

Ingredients:

8 cups sweet potatoes (about 4 large potatoes)
1 cup canned coconut milk (light or regular)
1/4 cup maple syrup
1/4 cup coconut oil, melted
1 Tbsp. ground flaxseed
1 tsp. vanilla
1 tsp. cinnamon
1/2 tsp. sea salt
1/2 tsp. freshly grated or ground nutmeg

Topping Ingredients:

1/2 cup brown sugar or coconut sugar
1/2 cup chopped pecans
1/3 cup gluten-free old-fashioned oats
1/3 cup gluten-free oat flour or almond flour
3-4 tbsps. coconut oil, in solid form

Directions:

1. Peel and chop the sweet potatoes into large chunks.
2. Place the chunks in a large saucepan and cover with cold water, bring to a boil and reduce to simmer. Simmer until the sweet potatoes are fork tender, about 15-20 minutes. Once done, drain well and let cool.
3. Meanwhile, preheat your oven to 350° and spray a little cooking spray on a 9x13 or 9x9 inch casserole dish.
4. In a mixing bowl, combine the pecans, oats, oat flour, and brown sugar. Cut in coconut oil with a fork or knife until the mixture is sandy with pea-sized chunks of oil. Set aside.
5. Place sweet potatoes into a large bowl and mash them with fork before adding coconut milk, maple syrup, oil, flaxseed, vanilla, cinnamon, nutmeg, and salt to the ball. Mix until everything is combined.
6. Spoon the sweet potato mixture into the prepared dish and sprinkle on the brown sugar and pecan mixture. Bake uncovered for 40-45 minutes, until the top is golden brown and the sweet potatoes are bubbling.

Gluten-free Cornbread

Ingredients:

1 1/2 cups gluten-free all-purpose flour
1 1/2 cups gluten-free cornmeal
1/3 cup sugar
2 tbsp. honey
2 tsp baking powder
1 tsp baking soda
1 tsp salt
2 eggs
1 1/2 cups milk
6 tbsp. unsalted butter
1 tsp bacon fat

Directions:

1. Preheat the oven to 200°C/400 degrees F.
2. Grease a medium-sized cast-iron skillet (or 8×8 baking dish) with bacon grease or butter, and place inside the oven while you prep the other ingredients.
3. In a large mixing bowl, add the flour, cornmeal, sugar, baking powder, baking soda, and salt. Whisk until well combined.
4. Melt the butter and let it cool slightly while you whisk together the eggs and milk in a separate bowl.
5. Once the butter is cool, add it to the wet ingredients.
6. Pour the wet ingredients into the dry and stir gently together with a wooden spoon or spatula. Don't over-mix, but let everything become incorporated.
7. Remove the heated skillet (or baking dish) from the ove and pour the batter in.
8. Turn the oven down to 350 degrees F and bake for 25-30 minutes, or until the top is brown and an inserted toothpick comes out clean.

Let cool slightly before slicing and serving.

Gluten Free Yellow Squash Casserole

Ingredients:

1/2 cup diced onion
1 tbsp. fresh thyme leaves, chopped
1 cup cooked brown rice
1 tbsp. extra-virgin olive oil
1 plum (Roma) tomato, diced
1/2 tsp. salt
1/8 tsp. pepper
1 medium zucchini, thinly sliced
1 medium yellow summer squash, thinly sliced
1/2 cup gluten-free shredded Italian cheese blend (2 oz.)

Directions:

1. Heat oven to 400 degrees F. Spray 1 1/2 to 2-quart shallow casserole (gratin dish) with cooking spray.
2. In small bowl, stir together onion, half of the thyme leaves, the rice, oil, tomato, 1/4 tsp. of the salt and the pepper.
3. Spoon into casserole; spread evenly. Alternately layer zucchini and squash, overlapping slightly, on top of rice mixture.
4. Sprinkle with remaining thyme and remaining 1/4 tsp. salt.
5. Cover; bake 20 minutes.
6. Sprinkle with cheese. Bake uncovered 10 to 12 minutes longer or until cheese is melted and starting to turn golden brown.
7. Cool 10 minutes before serving.

Gluten-Free Creamed Corn

Ingredients:

3 cups cooked sweet corn kernels
1/2 cup heavy cream
3 tbsps. butter
1 tsp. sugar
Salt and pepper, to taste

Directions:

1. Melt butter in large skillet over medium heat.
2. Add corn and stir to mix well. (If using frozen kernels, sauté until corn is thawed before adding other ingredients.)
3. Pour in heavy cream, sugar, salt and pepper. Continue cooking, stirring constantly, for about 10 minutes or until sauce is thick.

Gluten-Free Broccoli Casserole

Ingredients:

3 eggs
6 tbsps. gluten-free flour
2 cups frozen broccoli
1 lb cottage cheese
½ tsp. salt
2 cups cheddar cheese

Directions:

1. Beat the flour and eggs until smooth and then add the remaining ingredients.
2. Pour into a casserole dish, and bake uncovered at 350 for 70 minutes.
3. Let sit about 5 minutes before serving.

About the Author

Laura Sommers is **The Recipe Lady!**

She is a loving wife and mother who lives on a small farm in Baltimore County, Maryland and has a passion for all things domestic especially when it comes to saving money. She has a profitable eBay business and is a couponing addict. Follow her tips and tricks to learn how to make delicious meals on a budget, save money or to learn the latest life hack!

Visit her Amazon Author Page to see her latest books:

amazon.com/author/laurasommers

Visit the Recipe Lady's blog for even more great recipes and to learn which books are **FREE** for download each week:

http://the-recipe-lady.blogspot.com/

Subscribe to The Recipe Lady blog through Amazon and have recipes and updates sent directly to your Kindle:

The Recipe Lady Blog through Amazon

Laura Sommers is also an Extreme Couponer and Penny Hauler! If you would like to find out how to get things for **FREE** with coupons or how to get things for only a **PENNY**, then visit her couponing blog **Penny Items and Freebies**

http://penny-items-and-freebies.blogspot.com/

Other Books by Laura Sommers

- **Gluten Free Baking Recipes**

- **Gluten Free Cookie Recipes**

- **Gluten Free Cauliflower Recipes**

- **Gluten Free Cake Recipes**

- **Gluten Free Bread Recipes**

May all of your meals be a banquet
with good friends and good food.

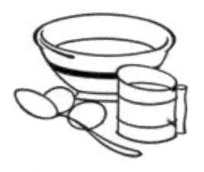